Meditation for Beginners:

Easy Guide to Begin Meditation

Table of Contents

Introduction

Chapter 1: What Is Stress?

Chapter 2: Why Meditate?

Chapter 3: Origins of Meditation

Chapter 4: Types of Meditation: Transcendental

Chapter 5: Types of Meditation: Heart Rhythm

Chapter 6: Types of Meditation: Kundalini

Chapter 7: Types Of Meditation: Guided Imagery

Chapter 8: Types Of Meditation: Qi Gong

Chapter 9: Types Of Meditation: Zazen

Chapter 10: Mindfulness Meditation

Chapter 11: Less-Traditional Meditation

Chapter 12: Meditation Best Practices

Chapter 13: 5-Minute Calming Meditation

Chapter 14: 30-Minute Complete Meditation

Conclusion

Introduction

Congratulations on downloading your personal copy of *Meditation for Beginners: Easy Guide to Begin Meditation.* Thank you for doing so.

The following chapters will discuss some of the many ways that meditation can reduce stress, improve your productivity and improve your life.

You will discover how important it is to practice meditation on a regular basis to get the full benefits. You will be glad you did!

There are plenty of books on this subject on the market, thanks again for choosing this one! Every effort was made to ensure it is full of as much useful information as possible. Please enjoy!

Chapter 1: What Is Stress?

In this age of modern technology and on-the-go attitude, stress is abundant. In general, stress is anything that creates a release of stress hormones within the body. It can be caused by just about anything, and for some people, just about everything. Stress is impossible to avoid and is a necessary, and sometimes good, part of life.

The stress reaction in the body is very complex, and for the sake of time, we will explain it simply. A stress response to something in the environment causes the body to release stress hormones, like cortisol and adrenaline. Their release causes blood pressure to rise, and blood and oxygen to flow to muscles among other things, to facilitate a 'fight or flight' situation. Basically, if we are threatened by something, our body becomes prepared to be assaulted or to flee from danger.

This chain of events was something the human body developed as a defense mechanism very early on in our history. As we evolved from lesser creatures, this one came with it. Back then, there were more physical threats to our existence than there are now. The threat of being attacked by a wild animal or by a tribe across the river required our bodies to be physically able to deal with that. When a threat is encountered, the body expands the totality of the hormones released, and when out of danger, returns to normal.

These days, there are many less physical threats to deal with as humans. For the majority of people, stress now comes from things like busy schedules, meeting deadlines and dealing with family issues. Unfortunately, the body does not know the difference and releases stress hormones as a response. Blood pressure rises, energy flows through you, and you feel anxious. This feeling often lasts because we are not expending the energy that has been created. Instead, we sit behind our desks or in our cars, letting that energy sit with us.

The result of this pent-up energy isn't good. It causes a number of physical and mental effects that are a detriment to good health and well-being. Some of the most common symptoms of stress are fatigue and headache. Another common symptom is stomach pain or indigestion. Long-term, people often develop irritable bowel syndrome (IBS), which can be primarily due to the stress response.

Feeling stressed ultimately wears us out much quicker and depletes our ability to think clearly as well. It also suppresses the immune system, meaning you are more susceptible to illnesses like cold and flu viruses. If you are feeling tired all the time, despite adequate sleep, stress hormones may be to blame.

While the acute symptoms are not so bad, the results of chronic stress can be drastic. Long-term chronic stress can lead to issues with high blood pressure, causes weight gain, hair loss and is a major cause of depression. If stress suppresses the immune system too much, it can actually trigger a number of autoimmune diseases, like lupus and multiple sclerosis (MS), as well as arthritis and thyroid problems.

To manage stress, it is important to know where it is coming from. It is not always possible to recognize all sources of stress, so you must do your best to deal with what you recognize. Take a good look at the following sources and determine where you should begin.

The most common cause of stress is work and career-related. It is true that you can't always pick your co-workers, and differences in opinion and work ethic are a common source of stress. You may not get along with everyone at work, but for stress relief, it is important to find common ground.

If it is not the people who surround you at work, it could be the work itself. If you are in a job that is unfulfilling and downright draining, stress is inevitable. It would be easy to recommend removing yourself from this terrible job, but that is not possible for most people. If you cannot get out, at least not right away, find the good parts of your job and focus on that. If you love your co-workers, focus on those great people to get through your day.

It is also important to think more long-term. If you would ultimately be happier making a career change, make moves to do that. Just the act of planning for your exit gives you hope and energy to deal with the stress of the job. One doesn't simply change careers, it involves a lot of thought. Start the planning process now and get excited!

Another common stressor is family life. Most Americans simultaneously work and look after a family and take care of a home. Regardless of your family structure, you must come home after work and clean the house, do laundry and make dinner. All of these things, after a long day at work, can be stressful and exhausting. Find ways to streamline your chores, get the whole family involved, and cut down on time.

While chores and daily tasks are unavoidable, bad relationships are. Perhaps it is family members, spouses, in-laws that stress you out. If you feel that a relationship you have is dysfunctional, or even mentally or verbally abusive, it is necessary to change it or remove yourself from the situation to reduce your stress. Carrying on with another person who has different opinions and dreams will inevitably end with a bit of conflict, and that is okay. Rather, it is how healthy your reaction and handling of the situation is that matters most.

No matter your type or level of stress, it is important to find ways to reduce it and relieve it when it happens. As our ancestors did, physical activity is a great way to reduce acute stress and jitters, but we must strive for better when dealing with chronic low-level stress. The answer to that is meditation.

Chapter 2: Why Meditate?

As we explained in Chapter 1, one of the answers to dealing with chronic stress is meditation. This is simply the process of straightening out your mind and logically assessing the situation to lower stress. There are many different types of meditation practices, which will be discussed in detail later in this book. If you are still stuck on the 'why?' of it, please continue reading.

According to a Harvard study, practicing meditation for just ten minutes every day reduces stress and lowers the chance of developing cardiovascular disease. Those are two major things. First, we already know that chronic stress is a precursor to many other health problems, including autoimmune disease and depression. The fact that cardiovascular health is improved is another big win. This is likely due in part to a more regulated blood pressure.

We discussed the carnal 'fight or flight' response in the previous chapter. The threat of danger causes a release of hormones that cause blood pressure to rise, the heart to beat rapidly and a number of other responses to prep the body to take action. Practicing meditation has actually been shown to have the opposite response, and the benefits of that are staggering.

Instead of raising the occurrence of common medical problems, it actually reduces them. How do just ten minutes of meditation per day have so much effect on our health? Let's take blood pressure as an example. If your blood pressure is slightly elevated above normal levels on a regular basis due to stress, ten minutes of relaxation could drop those levels below normal levels, to optimal. If a stressor is then added, it will likely only increase your blood pressure to normal levels.

Stress affects the body on a cellular level. Stress creates free radicals in the body, which age cells much quicker. In effect, if all of your cells are aging and turning over faster, it speeds up the aging process, as cells can only regenerate themselves a certain number of times. Once you hit that limit, there is no turning back.

This is the point at which collagen depletes in the skin causing wrinkles, and organ function decreases causing disease. The more stress you have, the faster this happens. They say stress causes wrinkles and gray hair, well, maybe that was quite literal. Don't think of meditation as just a way to reduce stress at the moment, but as a way to prolong your life and good health long term.

In addition, meditating gets your head in a better place to deal with stress in the first place. The mind is a busy place, dealing with thoughts of both the conscious and subconscious mind simultaneously, all day long. Meditation allows some of those open files to be dealt with and put away, leaving more energy to deal with the stress.

Regular meditation increases natural energy levels, leaving you more juice to deal with the daily grind. Imagine facing the day feeling like you've had a pot of coffee (minus the jitters), more alert and focused. This is possible, and without coffee, with the help of meditation.

For example, if you get to work already frazzled from your commute, how likely are you to snap at someone when they come to you with a problem? Would it be different if you had taken a few minutes in the parking lot to reset your mind before walking into work? Allowing meditation to get you in a good head space spares energy from being wasted in a negative way. Instead, you can focus on the good parts of your day, and deal with stress more productively.

The act of meditation also increases your productivity by focusing your mind and increasing your memory. Meditation recharges your batteries, allowing you to take on more work, and be more productive in smaller stretches of time. Perhaps you will find that a quick meditation session after lunch primes you for an afternoon of great energy and motivation.

All of this has a tremendous effect on mental health overall. Chronic stress is a cause of depression and anxiety, and people with a stressful job and life situations often fall victim to these problems. With regular meditation, it is possible to lift the spirits, better connect with your inner self, and find your purpose.

From the spiritual side of things, connecting with your inner self through meditation allows your inner guidance to reach your decluttered mind, guiding you where you need to go. Has anyone ever asked you a question you just couldn't answer? What would you do if you won the lottery? What job would you do if money was no object? If none of your current responsibilities existed, what would you focus your life on?

It is hard for a lot of people to answer these questions because they are so bogged down with the day to day grind that they forget who they are. Adding even a few meditative minutes to your day silences the constant asking of your surroundings and allows you to focus on you. Doing so brings you these answers in time.

If you were taken aback before by the idea of working toward your dream job, meditation is a great option for you. If you have no idea what that job would be, or that dream life would look like, you need to take time and really meditate on it. How sad would it be to realize that you did not live your best life when it was too late? Is that depressing? Anxiety-inducing?

How about money? Most people stress about paying bills and about making money. You can try all of the stress-relief programs and techniques out there, but none will work better than daily meditation. Even better, if you are on a budget, meditation is free!

There are a million reasons to meditate, but the only ones that matter are the ones that speak to you. Why not try meditation for a few days in a row and see how it impacts your day? Do you feel more in control of your emotions? More energized? Able to handle the stress of the day better? Most likely, you will see some good impact and decide that continued practice is warranted. After all, it's only ten minutes.

Keep in mind that meditation is only one key to reducing stress and creating a better quality of life. If, after meditation, you slip into bad habits, approach the day with a negative mindset and treat your body like a dump, then you will still have problems. Properly dealing with stress involves a transformation of life, mind, body, and soul.

Chapter 3: Origins of Meditation

Meditation is certainly nothing new. The earliest known practiced concept of meditation dates back to about 1500BC in early Hindu culture. The tradition of Vedantism was a common religion and spiritual practice in India at the time. This practice focused on liberating the inner spirit by gaining knowledge of the true identity.

Buddhist and Taoist religions were widely based on this early Hindu tradition. Like many religions, both ancient and modern focus on the idea of salvation. In Christianity, Judaism, and Islam, salvation often means worshipping a singular god and following the concepts of the holy books. Buddhism and similar religions and practices focus on salvation as well, but by finding one's true self and being at peace with the universe.

A scripture called the Bhagavad Gita was written around 300BC describing the different philosophies of meditation, and how to live in line with your spiritual essence. It states that all people have the ability to find a higher self through oneself, via the practice of meditation. More simply, you may find God, or a higher power, by recognizing your inner self through meditation.

It goes on to describe meditation as a means to be unscathed by the outer world. Someone who is at true peace will be unflustered by their surroundings. This sounds like the idea of stress reduction and higher tolerance for stress. This practice takes a great deal of concentration on behalf of the practitioner. Through this practice, the practitioner can find liberation.

Buddhism is practiced by some 500 million or more followers in the world today, and devout followers practice reading scriptures, denouncing unnecessary worldly things and practicing meditation. The Buddhist monk is often characterized as a man in a robe meditating in silence or taking a vow of silence. He often rids himself of physical things to reach a pure place. He is happy with himself.

Meditation has a very large part in that vision. Surely, not every Buddhist takes the practice to such lengths, but the bones are there. Following certain guidelines, moral rules and regular meditation are great ways to learn more about your inner self, to be respectful of your surroundings and the people around you, and to be an overall well-rounded person.

The ideas of meditation and finding salvation and bliss through the practice spread west during the early third century. At the time, Christianity was coming of age, and early adopters tried but did not see the wonder of meditation and related spiritual practices as beneficial.

The concept of Zen Buddhism soon followed and spread through Asia, becoming particularly popular in China. As the idea spread to new cultures, specific variations of practice developed that were unique to where it spread. In Japan, it was Japanese Zen and Seon Buddhism in Korea. Zen is all about self-control through meditation, which we will delve greater into in the following chapters.

During this time, the expansion of Buddhism and its offshoots did impact the west as well. There is evidence in the Torah showing that the patriarch Isaac may have done some sort of meditative practice throughout his story. Early Jewish practices focused on meditative prayer were evident. And, although true meditation did not take hold in the Christian religion, it is hard to ignore that repetitive prayers have a very meditative quality about them.

We also cannot ignore different styles of meditation used by cultures completely cut off from Asia during the expansion of Buddhism and meditation. Early Native Americans often held rituals that involved dancing and chanting as a way to center the mind and reach another spiritual plane. Groups of Native Americans as well as people of many cultures across the globe also facilitated reaching a meditative state with the use of mind-altering substances.

The main goal was to free the inner spirit to harness its knowledge. The interesting thing about the process of meditation, and these substances, is the physical effect on the body. Mind-altering drugs like those found in marijuana and acid have shown to affect the pineal gland, the spiritual third eye, a chakra renowned to be the center of spiritual awakening. Surely, it is possible to stimulate the third eye via meditation, but these substances seemed to be a more acute approach.

The idea of meditation evolved slowly over time, and today is practiced less for religious purposes, and more for the relaxation quality and stress reduction. In the 1920's Siddhartha, by Hermann Hesse was published, which was a chronicle of Buddha's life and spiritual journey. Although originally written in German, it took hold steadfast in the United States in the 1960's, shaping and solidifying meditation and yoga practices in the West. It is seen as a way to improve oneself, rather than a typical religion, although Buddhism and similar religions still exist today.

Practices like yoga also stemmed from the development of meditation. This is simply meditation in a more active form. While traditional meditation is done in solitude and stillness, yoga gets the entire body involved, moving energy around and creating a bigger sense of balance between body and mind.

No matter what style meditation you decide to practice, there is a common thread between all of them. The primary goal is to free your mind so that you may let your inner self guide you. The practice of meditation allows you to let go of worldly control through your logic mind, and take more guidance from your inner spirit, who is all-knowing and infinitely backs your cause. It does not matter whether or not you believe this on a religious level, the results are the same.

If you want to lead a more fulfilling, calm and balanced life, meditation is something you should try. The idea of practice is essential. One simply does not meditate once and unlock the secrets of the universe. It is a constant vigilance and search for inner peace that leads one to it. Take your time and really concentrate on what it is you wish to find, and you shall find it.

Take a look at the different offshoots of meditation outlined in the following chapters. Most likely, one practice or another will jump out at you as an obvious choice to follow. This could be your inner spirit jumping for joy, so go ahead and give in. It is totally fine to switch back and forth, or even mold some different techniques together. The goal is to find what works for you, and if that is a little bit of everything, varying day to day, that is your right.

Chapter 4: Types of Meditation: Transcendental

Transcendental meditation originated from Maharishi Mahesh Yogi, an Indian teacher who believed that meditating with a mantra was the most beneficial way to transcend to a higher conscious mind or place of being. Yogi was actually a modern-day pioneer in meditation, practicing his theories until his death in 2008.

Yogi brought his ideas from India to the United States in the 1960's. He didn't get the same welcome and respect as he did at home, and the practice really only took hold with a certain few, often labeled 'hippies', on the outskirts of society. The idea of said flower children to mainstream society at the time was a vision of groups of young people living in a van, hardly in touch with reality.

That idea is unfortunate, and for those mainstream followers that quietly practiced Yogi's teachings were the ones who really lived their best lives. And they still do. Many famous people, including Jerry Seinfeld and Oprah, practice Transcendental meditation. These seemingly well-adjusted, successful people could certainly give some credit to their practices.

Yogi believed that the world is in a state of stress and suffering. If he were alive today, he would probably still believe that. However, he also believed that it is possible for people to escape this reality by reaching within and harnessing the positive energy deep within themselves. The mind and spirit are always trying to find happiness, and the process of Transcendental meditation facilitates that much more quickly.

It seems natural that if the mind already shifts toward greater happiness, like molecules flow from most dense to less dense, simply allowing that to happen is the best way to be happy, enlightened even. Therefore, this practice does not require intense concentration, just the time and headspace to allow the mind to find happiness on its own.

The use of a mantra is helpful here because it gives the mind something to do. A mantra is simply a word, phrase or sound that implies a certain thought. If the mantra is a positive one, it sparks a chain of happy thoughts that start the brain off on a good note. It evokes nostalgia, happy times and situations.

A mantra can either be spoken aloud or repeated internally in silence. If you are a more visual person, you may find that concentrating on a physical picture or flicker of a candle flame is a more efficient way to focus your mind. This type of meditation requires no concentration or great effort, only the ability to focus attention on the mantra.

Practitioners can subscribe to Yogi's teachings and he recommends receiving a mantra from a trained teacher who has experience invoking suitable words that create the positive feelings. It is recommended to receive training from a skilled professional as there are seven steps to achieving the goals of Transcendental meditation. You are asked to meet with the professional for several sessions before you are given your mantra, which is yours and yours alone.

Reaching a state of bliss and transcendence is the ultimate goal. Those who regularly practice find themselves in a state of stillness and limbo. Their mind simply exists, it is at rest and in order. This state harnesses the infinite amount of energy stored within us and allows us to carry out our day drenched in that energy. Practicing this style of meditation once or twice a day is advisable to live a happy and fulfilled life on another plane.

Those not willing to go through formal training in Transcendental meditation still have the option to use mantras in their daily practices. If you do not feel ready to commit to such a practice, dig deep and try to find your own mantra that elicits a positive response. If there is a word or sound that always makes you happy or calm, try using that.

The testimonials are many, and always imply that regular Transcendental meditation is cause for increased productivity, less stress. It lowers blood pressure, supports the immune system and facilitates good habits that keep the body strong, like eating a proper diet, getting enough sleep and having the energy to exercise.

In the field of addiction recovery, Transcendental meditation is vital to keeping people sober. It allows the mind to focus on thoughts other than drugs or alcohol and gives people the strength and energy to focus on their long-term goals and stave off cravings.

Feelings are mixed in terms of mental health. Although meditation overall is thought to reduce anxiety and depression, the act of reciting and repeating a mantra is thought to create a mesmerized state, in which certain people with mental illness might lose themselves. However, there is no real evidence to back these claims up. Just a word of caution.

When it comes to your brain, Transcendental meditation has been shown to work the entire brain. It is thought that the entire brain works together during meditation, instead of just calling upon certain parts during normal thought patterns. The mind of a practitioner of Transcendental meditation is known to be sharper, and more able to handle complex tasks than the average person.

It is fine to be skeptical of such a seemingly-strange practice. What benefit could reciting a singular word or phrase every day really do for you? The answer is, you don't know until you try. Instead of being skeptical, try being curious and give it a try. You really have nothing to lose except for the stress and bonds of the current plane of energy you subscribe to.

Chapter 5: Types of Meditation: Heart Rhythm

Heart Rhythm Meditation is a more modern, scientific approach to traditional meditation. It was originally developed by Puran and Susanna Bair at the Institute for Applied Meditation. This method is a little more active than practices such as Transcendental Meditation and involved the concept of conscious breathing.

Conscious breath is rhythmic, such as the beat of your heart. The goal for this type of meditation is to sync the breath, heartbeat and circulatory system in an effort to calm nerves and reduce stress. This coordination happens by completing a series of breathing exercises.

The science behind this technique is rather interesting and has pause to back the ideas of meditation and relaxation as a whole. Studies have found that levels of carbon dioxide at the end of a breathing cycle are linked to heartbeat variability and frequency. When posed in a stressful situation, the heartbeat of a person who does not exercise regular meditation is quite varied and irregular. That of a practiced meditator is balanced and rhythmic. More irregularity in the frequency of heartbeat is linked to medical problems like heart disease.

This heartbeat variability is directly affected by the breath, and by exercising certain breathing patterns, we can manipulate heartbeat variability. These studies also show that such breathing techniques also lower the average heart rate as well, a classic sign of good cardiovascular health. This is similar to the heartbeat being lower in a person who exercises regularly. Strictly as a medical approach, this helps prove that meditation is tangibly beneficial to health.

There are many stages of heart rhythm meditation, and the first is concentration. Just like other forms of meditation, we must concentrate on something to focus our minds. In this case, focus on your heart. It helps to place your hand over your heart or a pulse point to recognize the beat. As you sit calmly, start timing your breathing with this beat. Do not try to breathe for each beat, as you will hyperventilate. Simply notice the natural rhythm of your breath against the beat, maybe every 4 beats you complete the cycle. Regiment your breath to sync with the beat.

This stage alone is very beneficial for monitoring stress levels throughout the day. This exercise can be done at any time, and if you notice that you are suddenly breathing one breath for every 8 heartbeats, you know it is elevated, and you are stressed. You can then take steps to slow the breath in an effort to slow the heart back to normal.

The second stage of Heart Rhythm meditation is contemplation. You must be aware of the connection of your heart and breath, both physically and emotionally. Becoming more aware that energy and electricity flow between these organs, and between your heart and the hearts of others gets you thinking more compassionately, empathetically and charismatically.

The final stage is the actual meditation practice. This is the part where you sit quietly and reflect. Realize in this moment of sync that you are a part of everything, and everything is part of you. It is all connected, and love, peace, and joy live in your heart.

Let's take a look at some of the breathing exercises that will be helpful to this practice. Remember that the idea is to consciously change your breath so that you fully inhale and exhale, releasing any carbon dioxide that has stagnated in your lungs. This act alone allows for more oxygen to flow in, increasing your energy and adding some pep to your step.

Before getting started, find a quiet, comfortable seated position. Posture is important here because being slumped over means you won't be able to get all of your air in and out. Sit up straight and tall and allow your airways to open all the way to the corners of your lungs.

To begin, just take note of your breath. Notice the normal patterns, how long you remain still between each inhale and exhale. As you practice at different times, you will notice different types of breath. Get comfortable and familiar with these changes before moving on in your practice.

Next, it is time to take control of the breath. Try to inhale for as much time as you exhale, steady in and out. Try to gain balance. Breathe with as little sound or interruption as possible. Your breath should be smooth. As you breathe, imagine the air pulsing in and out of your heart area.

Soon after, consciously give a full exhale on each breath. Leave no molecule of carbon dioxide in those lungs. Use your abdominal muscles to push up and out. Do not linger in this state, breathe in immediately to avoid the need for gasping breath. Notice how energized this inhale breath feels after the long exhale.

Try the same with your inhalation, filling your lungs as if they feel about to burst, then swiftly exhale, relieving that tension and pushing out any negative energy and emotions within you. As you repeat these breathing patterns, try different variations, like the ones below, to enter different states of focus and consciousness.

The 'swinging breath' is a common practice and is a simple 1:1 inhale to exhale pattern. Simply breathe in for a count of 8, then out for a count of 8. This long count allows all of the carbon dioxide out, as at the last breath, you will be pushing every last bit out.

The 'square breath' is a great exercise to reduce stress and anxiety. In reality, any act of conscious breathing distracts the mind from stress, but the staggered breath of square breathing really seems to do the trick. Here, breath in for a count of 8, hold it in for 16 counts, then exhale for 8 counts. Envision oxygen coming in on the first 8, that oxygen collecting all of the negative energy as you hold your breath, and all of that negativity exiting your body as you exhale for 8 counts. Repeat a few times, or until your anxiety has calmed.

Any time you stagger your breathing, there is the chance of getting a little light-headed, especially when you are holding your breath. Ideally, you will do this in a seated position, somewhere quiet where you can focus. Be sure to monitor how you are feeling and stop if you begin to feel dizzy. As you are changing the way your heart beats, although in a positive way, it is important to check with your doctor to get clearance, just to be safe.

Overall, this form of meditation is great for beginners, and for those who have a hard time focusing their meditative practice. The act of conscious breathing gives the mind something to focus on, which may be easier than practices that simply allow thoughts to flow in and out of the mind. For some of us, this enlightenment only lasts a fleeting moment, as the mind wanders quickly.

Chapter 6: Types of Meditation: Kundalini

Kundalini is described as the energy that is coiled and gathered along the base of the spine. The ultimate goal of Kundalini meditation is to awaken this energy, which is thought to be a powerful source of creativity and infinite wisdom. It is almost always thought about as feminine in nature. In writing, Kundalini is often depicted by a snake coiled around three and one-half times along the base of the spine.

Unlike the well-documented third eye, which in a physical sense relates to the pineal gland, resting safely between the hemispheres of the brain, Kundalini is not something that is tangible. It is simply a guiding energy that exists but is not tied down to a physical structure.

Kundalini is the energy of the entire body. It tends to center and collect itself around the seven main chakras in the body. This energy lies dormant, and the ultimate benefit of practicing Kundalini meditation is to awaken that energy.

How can we awaken Kundalini? The most beneficial practice to mobilizing this energy is yoga. Several teachers caution not to try to awaken Kundalini without the guidance of a true Master. Once Kundalini is awakened, she will transcend the chakras all the way to your mind. Her infinite wisdom and clarity will begin to awaken thoughts and feelings in you that you are not ready for.

The general recommendation is to be in a good mental state before conjuring this energy. If you have not dealt with the traumas and hardships of your life, you may suddenly be overcome with emotions as Kundalini is awakened inside of you. This energy will force you to recognize and confront all of your past discord. Of course, this sense of self-realization is really a good thing, but only if you are ready for it.

There may be physical ramifications too. The Kundalini Support Organization states that people often experience muscle spasms, hot flashes, and nerve sensations, along with digestive issues and triggering latent disease. These symptoms are thought to be Kundalini's way of ridding the body of negative energy. While these side effects may be a turn-off, we need to look at what is happening behind the scenes.

The energy of Kundalini is of infinite wisdom, therefore, when it is awakened, you will begin to experience life from her all-knowing angle. You will never experience the same thoughts and feelings again. What do you have to gain? Hopefully, a new sense of understanding within the universe that can guide you to your true destiny. For many, this involves a complete upheaval of life as they know it.

Kundalini is priming you to accept greater amounts of energy, Prana, from the universe. Doing so will make you feel more alive, more intense and passionate about things. You will love on a whole new level, and understand the workings of the universe like you never have. Once you have awakened Kundalini, there is no going back.

Given all of these warnings, it is important to note that Kundalini meditation should not be the first type of meditation tried, especially if you are new to the concept. The good news is, there is a great deal of concentration and focus required to awaken Kundalini. Most beginners do not possess this skill, as their meditation practice is just beginning. Once you have mastered other forms of meditation and have reached a peak benefit, it could be time to try this.

So, if you are ready for it, how do we awaken her? There are three phases that are meant to awaken Kundalini. The first is diaphragmatic deep breathing in meditation. The purpose of training your diaphragm is to have the ability to regulate your breathing and bring you back to center.

To get started, extend your stomach, pushing it as far out as you inhale as possible. When you exhale, push your stomach muscles further, allowing every last breath to escape. This exercise strengthens the diaphragm muscles. Practicing this technique often throughout the day, and during your practice may leave your muscles aching, a sign of a truly good workout.

To extend this workout further, use cyclic breathing like we discussed in Transcendental meditation. A series of counts in a 1:1 inhale to exhale is beneficial, but also try 4 counts in and 2 counts out, or four in, four to hold, and four out. In the short term, this type of work awakens some energy and makes concentration and focus sharper.

As you practice, you will be able to take more air in with each breath. No more shallow breathing, but full, oxygen-rich breaths. As this is the same concept as in Transcendental meditation, we can expect a certain level of breath and heartbeat sync as well. This will then allow you to control your heartbeat. This is step number two.

The backward-flowing method is the third step to Kundalini awakening. This is the idea that we can draw up primal energy from Kundalini to the brain. There are many explanations of it, all of which involve harnessing energy from deep within, sometimes equating to sexual energy, and using it to fuel the brain in the process of self-actualization. Basically, you are asking energy to flow backward, up the spine, to the brain.

It is recommended to seek help and guidance from a Master in this process, and outside of these professionals. There is not much clear-cut guidance available. To begin, take a comfortable seated position. Keep your posture aligned properly and feel the air inhale and exhale from your belly region. As you breathe in, your lower belly inflates and deflates as you exhale your breath.

Once your diaphragm is working, you will feel a build up of energy in your lower belly, and a tingle in the base of your spine. Direct your energy to switch directions, mentally pulling energy up the spine. Imagine it, and feel it happening. You will begin to sense the energy movement, at which point it is in your mind.

Reaching awakened Kundalini will take quite a bit of practice and concentration. One does not simply meditate in this way for ten minutes and expect it to happen. If you are truly interested in reaching a new level of consciousness in your meditation practice, focus on awakening Kundalini. Give it time and be patient with the results. You will know it when it happens.

Chapter 7: Types Of Meditation: Guided Imagery

Guided imagery is a great meditation practice for those just getting started with meditation. The goal of most types of meditation is to focus the attention of the mind inward, casting out all thoughts and emotions related to external triggers. The benefits are great for stress reduction and mental clarity. Unfortunately, we are so overstimulated by our external lives, that we often lose our inner selves in them.

For a beginner, it can be very difficult to harness this focus, and so practices like guided imagery or the use of sounds like gongs can help draw the attention of the mind away from its humdrum thoughts and draw it to some inner thinking. The mind likes to work, and sometimes it takes some coaxing to get it to sit down and relax.

Guided imagery meditation is a method that often involves an instructor and pupil. The pupil is you and your busy mind. The instructor is trained to deliver an image to you, something that you can focus on, through speech. The instructor will describe a scene, often something soothing and calming, down to the last detail. The mind easily becomes compelled to hear the story and to imagine every last bit of information in the mind.

Depending on the level of practice, this form of meditation can be synonymous with hypnosis. Once a person is in a deep state of relaxation and fully engulfed in the scene, the practitioner can instill positive words and manipulate thought patterns. Of course, these should all be positive affirmations and thoughts created by a responsible party.

It is not simply a collection of sights, it involves every sense in your body. Proper guided imagery has you seeing the place, hearing sounds associated with it, feeling the air on your face, the ground underfoot, and smelling the flowers, the salt air, whatever the case may be. Engulfing all the senses really brings the mind to a state of relaxation as if you were really there.

This is an all-inclusive act for the brain. It takes analytical and creative power to form such an image in your mind. It requires the left and right sides of your brain to function and act together, and there is no room for other thought. This type of meditation is great because it does not require a tremendous amount of focus to get started, and it works those creative mind muscles to become more able to focus on the future.

Guided imagery meditation can be used for a number of purposes, and the outcome is directly affected by what type of image is used for the practice. The most common use is for stress reduction and relaxation. An image of a calm meadow or a warm beach elicit feelings of calm and collection. A simple ten-minute guided session can lower blood pressure, calm racing thoughts and reduce anxiety.

If this is your goal, getting started with guided meditation is easy. You can certainly try to find a practitioner in your area to help you get started. If you are lacking a professional, or simply do not feel comfortable seeking one, there are many online resources with videos and soundtracks of guided imagery.

If you are truly ready, you can even guide it for yourself, however, you will be prone to your own thoughts and feelings. Sure, you can imagine a beach somewhere, but it may be easier to let go if you take yourself out of that creative process. The act of being guided by something outside of yourself facilitates the meditation process. Otherwise, you are still subject to your own thoughts and feelings.

This can be done just about anywhere. All it requires is a quiet space, a computer if you are using a video or soundtrack, and your mental focus. Simply sit quietly, listen or watch, and concentrate on the task at hand. Do your best to flush out wandering thoughts and give a good effort to simply focus on what you are supposed to be focused on.

Guided imagery can also be a means of therapy, and is actually catching on in terms of emotional healing from traumatic events and addictions. A trained therapist can use guided imagery to help a patient with emotional trauma and to reduce anxiety. For example, let's say the patient is afraid of hcights. While this may be the least of their problems, it is a tangible example.

In this case, the practitioner can have the patient imagine that they are atop a high-rise building. As the image is clearly imagined in their mind, their blood pressure begins to rise and they get anxious. At this point, the practitioner can talk the patient through calming themselves and realizing the situation for what it is. As long as they are not out on the ledge, they are safe. There is no danger, and the reaction is simply a figment of their imagination.

This practice allows a practitioner to help a patient face their fears, reduce anxiety and heal, all within the comforts of their office. It does not require the therapist to join the patient on the roof or experience the physical or emotional trauma with them. This practice works wonders for people with social anxiety as well. The patient can imagine navigating being out in public and conversing with people, learning to self-soothe and calm their fears.

The practice is also great for dealing with substance abuse and addiction, as these are mostly emotional problems too. Substance abuse often stems from anxiety, both social and situational. Alcohol or drugs can be a way to self-soothe. A practitioner can invoke a stress-inducing scene, then teach the patient to self-soothe in more productive ways, instead of reaching for their vice.

No matter the use, guided imagery has been shown to reduce blood pressure, cholesterol and blood sugar levels in patients. It can boost the immune system and improve healing. Curiously, it also enhances physical and mental performance, allowing people to master complex skills and lower anxiety in events like test-taking and public speaking.

People have been known to quit smoking or even lose weight after proper guided imagery. If you think the mind cannot be manipulated, you are wrong. As a final note, make sure your source of guided imagery is a responsible party.

Chapter 8: Types of Meditation: Qi Gong

Qi Gong, or 'energy techniques' is a series of practices that predate recorded history. 'Qi' stands for breath, and is often associated with creativity, function and overall consciousness. 'Gong' stands for practice. This practice of health and wellness combines meditation, breathing practices and movement to promote overall health and well-being. Mindfulness also plays an important role and is crucial to recognize your body and mind in any given movement.

Practicing Qi Gong puts you in a relaxed and renewed state. Regular practice brings energy and life to your immune system and keeps the flow of energy circulating around the body. It helps bring necessary oxygen and nutrients to cells in the body, increasing metabolism, speeding the healing process and managing your mood. Just about anyone can practice Qi Gong because the movements can be done sitting, standing or lying down.

The practice of Qi Gong breaks down to three Intentful Corrections, which are adjusting the posture, breathing, and control of the mind. It originated in ancient China and was created to promote good health, emotional well-being, and connection to the spirit. The practices are still part of Chinese medicine to this day. The movements and postures along with specific breathing patterns get energy flowing in the body. It is similar to yoga, and it is often called movement meditation.

Regular practice of Qi Gong is thought to extend life and

improve quality of life for much longer than the average person. Nearly two-thirds of disease inflicted on humans these days are preventable. Taking action and practicing energy movements like the ones in Qi Gong helps alleviate disease.

There are many different types of Qi Gong, many which will look familiar. Tai Chi is commonly practiced in this day and age. This, and most types of Qi Gong can be done by most people because it is low impact, and does not require a great exertion of energy, as in most popular exercise. Poses are relatively easy to maneuver, and when paired properly with breath work, are beneficial to all.

The poses and breath work also promote good posture and balance. As we age, it is important to maintain these things to stay active and healthy well into our years. People who move more often are less likely to have falls creating injuries, a common pitfall for older people.

Qi Gong works so well because it promotes the stimulation of the lymphatic system. This organization of glands helps remove toxins from the body, collecting them in lymphatic ducts. Blood does not commonly flow through these areas and collections of toxins often build up in the lymph system. The series of movements associated with Qi Gong helps to flush out these ducts and clear toxins out of the body. This is thought to be a major advantage to the immune system and prevents acute illness and chronic disease.

The great thing about Qi Gong is that it is an active form of meditation. For people that tend to need something to do and get distracted by more formal meditation, Qi Gong is a great option. Following instructions and patterns helps keep the mind focused while meditating at the same time. Getting movement involved is a great way to connect body and mind, and get a good work out at the same time. The more you stay focuses on the practice, the more meditative the session will be.

If you are new to Qi Gong, it can certainly help to learn the ropes at a formal class. Qi Gong and Tai Chi are relatively common, so it should not be a problem to find a class in your area. Be sure to wear comfortable clothes that you can move in.

Spontaneous Qi Gong may be a good place to start as well, although it may feel a little silly, to begin with. Spontaneous Qi Gong is simply the act of moving your body in any which way it pleases. Simply move in which way your body compels you. For beginners, this may be a little difficult, as your mind is not open to connect to your body in such a way. However, you can easily change this idea and be open to a sort of Qi Gong dance of your own creation. If you are a little self-conscious, don't be afraid. Chinese practitioners have often thought of rhythmic movement and shaking as a form of illness-eliminating therapy for centuries.

More formal classes will teach you about how different movements correspond to Yin and Yang, or negative and positive, light and dark. The idea is to create balance and harmony within the body, and you must tailor your movements to Yin and Yang.

Is it possible to attain true enlightenment through Qi Gong? Yes! The natural flow of movement and energy throughout the body can easily be described as a meditative experience. As many cultures look to dance and rhythmic movement to create a trance-like state, so too is Qi Gong. This form of meditation can certainly create the enlightenment you seek.

If you feel you would like to begin Qi Gong as a practice, start with a few basic movements. Simply take a few minutes to just swing back and forth. Stand tall, and move your hips and torso so you gently sway your upper body left and right. Let your arms swing gently by your sides. Close your eyes and engulf yourself in the rhythm of it. Continue for a few minutes and recognize how relaxed and lulled you become by this.

Allow your mind to calm and focus only on this movement, and sync your breath with the steady movement. Simply be mindful of the movements you are making. Keep your shoulders in a natural, comfortable slump. Do not focus on maintaining strict posture, just do what is comfortable.

This simple movement will give you a good idea of the effects of Qi Gong. There are, of course, many poses and actions to practice for Qi Gong, and the results will bring energy to your body, reduce anxiety and blood pressure and give you a clarity you may not have felt before. Make a point to practice for just ten or fifteen minutes per day and start reaping the benefits of Qi Gong.

Chapter 9: Types of Meditation: Zazen

Zen is a common term we use to describe something or someone as relaxed, cool and still. We hear of Zen gardens, which are meant to be places for relaxation and reflection. Zen was originally an offshoot of Buddhism which focuses solely on the practice of meditation. In Japanese, Zen is a path to enlightenment, one of which was completed by Buddha.

Zen is practiced to open the mind to its true self, a spirit of love and compassion. This practice was thought to be the true path of enlightenment, removing the need for tangible scriptures and formal religious practices as they were known in their time. Another common concept in the religion of Zen Buddhism was the idea that living an impoverished life was the only way to recognize what is truly important in the world: the inner self and intangible things like spirit and wisdom. Tangible things just get in the way.

Zazen is the meditation piece of the Zen Buddhist movement. It is the very heart of Zen itself, and many schools were dedicated and still are centered on this practice. The idea of this meditation as Buddha put it was to forget yourself in your meditation so that you could truly enlighten yourself and connect with the energy of the universe.

Zazen is practiced in a seated position, as is often depicted in pictures and sculptures of Buddha. Sitting on the floor helps ground your energy, making it much easier to connect and concentrate on the positive energy given to you by the earth. If this doesn't feel quite right, try sitting on a small pillow, allowing your knees to face downward and even touch the ground. This method of meditation is very easy to practice, so long as you can sit quietly and take time to reflect inwardly on yourself.

The goal of Zazen is to focus and sync the body, mind, and breath altogether. The first step is to pay attention to the body. As you sit quietly, simply feel your body. Feel that your bottom is rooted to the floor. Feel the back of your hands touch your knees as your palms face the sky. Feel the rise and fall of your belly as you breathe in and out. Feel the energy flowing through every inch of you.

Once you have recognized your body and the energy flowing through it, focus in on your breath. Breathe in through your nose, keeping your mouth closed. Keep your tongue pressed against the top of your mouth. You may keep your eyes open but focus your gaze downward. Tuck your chin in a little, allowing your head to face downward.

Focus on your current breath. It should be slow and steady. A quick and shallow breath is indicative of stress and disharmony. Focus on steadying the breath, slowing it down. Breathe from your hara, a spot just above the navel. Feel energy build there and take each breath from it. Begin counting your breath. Count each inhale and exhale cycle up to ten times. See if you can focus your mind on this process for the full count of ten. If you cannot, start over and continue this practice until you have focused your mind on the task for at least ten counts.

This practice focuses the mind and sharpens your awareness. The goal is to stop the background chatter going on in your subconscious so that you may focus on what is going on n the forefront. If the mind is not divided thinking of too many things at once, it will be focused enough to do really well at the one task you are truly focused on.

After you feel that the attention has focused, forego the counting and simply allow your breathing to return to normal, with no strict in and out. At this time, your mind will be relaxed, and you are in a deeper meditative state. In this state, random thoughts will flow into your headspace. Simply allow them to be, but do not attach any emotion or action to the thought. Just let each one enter and leave in due course.

As your mind wanders more, bring it back to center by practicing the counting ritual again. Each time you cycle through this pattern, you enter a deeper and deeper state of meditation. At full Zazen, you may only breathe a few times each minute. Your breath and your mind are connected. When you are breathing infrequently, it means that your mind is in a deep state of relaxation.

Like any form of meditation, Zazen requires practice and dedication. You simply cannot reach a full state of enlightenment unless you commit to practicing this form of meditation on a regular basis. Doing so will reduce your overall stress level and incorporate peace and calm into your daily life. You will soon find that you cannot live your life without it.

Chapter 10: Mindfulness Meditation

Mindfulness meditation is another great way to introduce yourself to the practice of meditation. All you need is a comfortable seat, a bit of focus and a steady breath to practice. It does not require knowledge of specific breathing techniques, and you just need to be in the moment while it is happening.

The idea of mindfulness certainly isn't new, and there are applications all over the realm of wellness. Eating mindfully means we are taking care to recognize each bite of food, tasting it for what it is and feeling its impact on our bodies. Being mindful in everyday activities means appreciating the little moments that make up our day, instead of rushing through and missing all of the simple pleasures.

The same concept applies in mindfulness meditation. In fact, it is simply being with your body, in the stillness of your mind in the moment of meditation that defines mindfulness meditation. The stigma about meditation is that the outcome will be enlightenment. We often put too much pressure on the anticipated end result to really get anything good out of meditation. In fact, many people stop because the long-term effects don't seem to be what they expected.

The idea of mindfulness meditation is to simply appreciate and accept the practice of meditation for what it is at that given moment. The meditation process itself is of value, not just the resulting sense of calm thereafter.

To practice mindfulness meditation, simply find a nice quiet, warm room where you can sit and relax. Leave your phone and other electronics outside, as you are simply here to be in the moment. Sit comfortably, with your back straight and legs crossed. Do not stiffen the spine, just find a comfortable, upright position. Place your hands on top of your legs, with your upper arms by your side. Do not slouch over. Let your gaze fall slightly to the ground.

Call your attention to your breath. Feel the oxygen rush into your lungs as it enters your body. Feel the carbon dioxide rush back out as you push that air out. Imagine that the air has a certain glimmer, and imagine it swirling around, sparkling and glowing through the inside of your lungs. Simply be there in the moment, taking gratitude for your breath.

Follow that breath outside of the lungs. Imagine the oxygen flowing from the lungs to your bloodstream, quickly pulsing throughout the body bringing energy and light to every tissue and cell you have. Inevitably, your mind will lose focus on the sensations of your breath, and other thoughts may cloud your space. Don't beat yourself up, this is natural.

Instead of forcibly trying to push the thought out, embrace it for a quick moment, recognize that it is there, but do not assign any value to it. Think of that thought as a paper airplane. See that it is there, a piece of folded white paper, and then send it sailing on its way. No judgments, and no expectations to deal with the thought as it passes through.

Depending on your time constraints, it may be a good idea to set aside a designated amount of time for this practice. If you plan to meditate until you have come to some epiphany, it puts too much pressure on the practice. Instead, plan to dedicate ten or fifteen minutes to your practice and even set a timer. Be happy with the progress and clarity you have made in that time and go on about your day.

After your practice, you will find a bit more clarity and mindfulness rubbing off on your daily tasks. The practice of mindfulness illuminates multiple portions of the brain at one, allowing your analytical and creative mind to function as one. This hardly ever happens in the grand scheme of things. We often have either logical thought or creative thought. Most times, the logical, day to day operator side of your brain wins out, and your creativity gets stuffed in a corner. By activating this center of your brain, it allows you to think differently going forward.

To keep up these feelings, practice mindfulness meditation on a daily basis. Between those sessions, practice being mindful in your everyday life. Take a quick timeout a few times a day to stop and take in where you are and what you are doing. Appreciate it for what it is. Even if you are in the middle of a stressful meeting, you can be mindful and appreciative of the fact that you have a job at all.

This stress is a sign that you are pushing forward and are being an active participant in your life. Leave the stress behind and move on with the day. Avoid getting back on autopilot and allowing your mind to wander and rest as you function in daily life Be aware of what you are doing at all times.

Chapter 11: Less-Traditional Meditation

There are many different offshoots of meditation. Finding something that works for you is just a part of the meditation process. It is important to consider, however, that traditional meditation doesn't work for everyone. Not everyone buys into the notion of sitting calmly or practicing specific movements and breathing patterns to reach a place of enlightenment. Really, meditation refers to any practice that puts your mind in a Zen place, no matter how unorthodox.

For a lot of people, meditation comes in the form of exercise. Sure, yoga and Qi Gong are forms of exercise, but runners, swimmers, and weightlifters often say that they get a sense of peace, calm and control over their lives when they exercise. Any exercise can give this effect, but there is something about the repetitive motions of running or any monotonous movement that creates a trance-like state.

Consider running, for example. Just about anyone can gather the strength to run a short distance It is another thing completely to run a long distance, like a marathon. You can practice and condition your body to be up to the challenge, but the real challenge of a long run is mental.

It takes a great deal of focus to convince yourself to keep running, even when the body is telling you to stop. After a few miles, begin counting your steps or pacing your breathing with every step you take. The sensation of your feet hitting the pavement below you sinks into every bone and fiber of your being. You are totally committed to the movement, to the point when your mind doesn't think about much else.

For others, the quiet-time associated with a run is what helps them navigate thoughts and feelings to bring about a sense of calm. Ideally, the goal of meditation is to eliminate all thought and be at one with your inner self, however, the process of rationalizing disturbing thoughts and coming to terms with problems is a huge step for reaching your enlightenment.

Other physical exercises, like weight lifting, can have the same meditative qualities. Weightlifters, for example, count their repetitions, focusing on proper form and muscle feeling, leaving little room for random thoughts to enter their headspace. It gives them a chance to relax and unwind, forgetting the troubles of the day.

Meditation can be facilitated by things like heat. People often partake in saunas to help rid the body of toxins, but it also brings calm and focus to the mind. Extreme heat, like that of a sauna, causes the mind to focus on steadying the breath and maintaining a safe core temperature. In practices like Bikram yoga, a trance-like state often occurs because the mind is so hyper-focused on steadying the breath and remaining cool that it literally cannot think of anything else. This really allows you to sit with yourself and simply be in the moment.

Some use aromatherapy as a means of relaxation as well. Certain essential oils, like lavender and mint, are calming and energizing. The simple act of smelling these oils brings a sense of calm. Smell has often been something of a question in the medical field. Certain smells can bring out memories and elicit emotional and physical responses. For example, if maple syrup reminds you of a time you ate pancakes with your grandmother, smelling syrup could bring back those good feelings. It is no wonder then, that certain smells and oils can have a therapeutic, calming effect on the brain.

Music is another great escape for the mind. Focusing on and listening to different kinds of music brings out the creative side of the brain, allowing it to focus in on the melody, rather than that stack of paperwork on your desk. Different types of music elicit different types of responses, and certain singers, styles of music, and even sound level will give you different meditative results. This is most like guided imagery, where you are susceptible to influence by an outside party.

People often say that heavy metal and rap are inflammatory types of music in that either the lyrics or the music are offensive to the ear and elicit a negative response. Then again, those that love the music perceive it as an outlet for their negative feelings, and the idea that they can relate to the music is therapeutic.

In general, rocking out to some calming, soothing music generally brings about a Zen state. If that isn't your thing, at least make a point to listen to songs that remind you of good times and happy memories to draw out good emotions to soothe your stress.

There really is no wrong way to meditate. Do whatever is

necessary to reach a state of calm and relaxation. Just remember that there is always more that could be gained if you branch out and try different modes of meditation. While music or exercise may speak to you, so may a more formal method of meditation. You certainly won't know until you try, and you have nothing to lose.

Chapter 12: Meditation Best Practices

No matter what type of meditation you subscribe to, make sure to practice in a way that is beneficial for your everyday life. By following the guidelines listed below, you can create a habit of daily meditation that will guide your life and awaken your inner spirit. Doing so will put you in better touch with your deepest needs and desires.

First, make sure you are doing something daily. As was the case with scientific evidence for Transcendental meditation, experts found that each meditation session lowered blood pressure to astoundingly low levels, and maintaining daily practice kept them there. The same subjects also reported feeling less stressed and more able to deal with the problems of daily life.

Therefore, it is better to practice for just a short time every day, rather than for a large block of time once in a while. Instead of dedicating your Sunday to meditation, spread the wealth throughout the week to keep your head straight and your spirit front and center. That great feeling meditation brings will likely only last until Monday at lunchtime.

Next, try to dedicate a specific place and time to your practice. In starting any habit, it is important to specify where and when you plan to do something. Having a flexible timeline will often mean doing it late, which turns into doing it never.

Start your practice small. Your daily habit does not necessarily mean taking an hour at the end of the day to light candles, play music and be at one with yourself. It could simply mean taking ten or fifteen conscious minutes as you crawl into bed to focus and quiet your mind before bed. In fact, this could be a great place to start. Meditation is great for priming the mind for sleep. As you meditate before bed, you may be getting a better night's sleep in the process. This could snowball into a better, more productive day tomorrow.

As you are beginning your practice, it may take longer to reach a meditative state. It is only human to let our minds wander. Instead of beating yourself up about it, just accept it as a state of your consciousness. Forgive yourself, as you are just beginning your practice, and it should not be expected to be perfect now, if ever. Begin by practicing more forgiving forms of meditation like mindfulness or guided meditation. This allows less stress on the brain and gives it something to do, instead of forcing it to suddenly come to terms with its existence.

Another great practice to try when starting out is keeping a meditation journal. Writing your thoughts and feelings down can be therapeutic and life-altering in itself. However, the idea of writing just a few adjectives down describing your mood or state of mind prior to and after meditation may help you see the impact. You may also choose to write about which methods help you reach a quieter state of mind with greater ease. Reflect on your journal writing often to stay active in the process, and to determine what practices work for you.

The most important aspect of any meditation practice is to keep an open mind. If you go into a meditation session half expecting to fail and not reach a state of well-being, you are manifesting your own destiny. If you got a little scared reading the section on Kundalini and now fear what might happen if she is awakened, you are closing your spirit in.

Keep in mind that your inner spirit knows no time or space boundaries. It simply is, and it is only harnessed by the closed mind. Instead of being afraid of what will happen, try being open-minded and curious about the possibilities that await you. You may find your path to enlightenment is a little bumpy, but if you truly wish to transform your life and mind, you need to be prepared for some change.

This may mean a bit of physical change, a different outlook on relationships and career choices, or it may just mean that you go about your same activities with a new attitude and sense of appreciation. No matter what comes about, just be open to it. Remember that your inner spirit is all-knowing and always has your best interests in mind. If you trust that it is guiding you in the right direction, and if you trust that you are reading its signals properly, you ultimately cannot fail. However, sometimes making it to a glorious place means being dragged through the mud first.

Chapter 13: 5-Minute Calming Meditation

The purpose of a short meditation session is to bring about an immediate sense of calm. Try this routine any time you feel acutely stressed or fatigued. This routine will help calm your nerves and re-energize your spirit to tackle the rest of your day.

Find a calm spot to escape for a few minutes. This could mean shutting your office door at work, taking a few minutes in the bathroom away from the family, or just taking a quick walk around the block.

Of course, getting to a meditative state in a very short five-minute window can be difficult, so we will impart the ideas of guided imagery to facilitate a quick transition to meditation. Enjoy!

Find yourself in a quiet space, even if it is only a radius of five feet from the nearest external stimulation. Imagine that an orb of quiet is surrounding your entire body. Gather it in your heart space. As you breathe in and out, feel the energy building in your heart. Once it feels big enough, push it outward. Imagine it radiating from every inch of your skin. Feel it gather around you, creating a bubble that encapsulates your entire body.

Take a moment to feel the energy that surrounds you, loud and present, yet calming and quieting as it drowns out the noise and chatter around you. Take in a deep breath, pulling some of that special energy back in toward you. Breathe deep, pulling inward until it feels as if you could not take another breath.

Hold that breath there for a second, feeling its weight within your chest. Imagine that the oxygen is flowing through your lungs, reaching every cell. As the air delivers oxygen, so too is it also gathering all of the stress and negative energy you are currently feeling.

Exhale slowly, yet forcefully, pushing every ounce of negativity harnessed within you. Feel and see it exiting your body, escaping from your capsule of energy out into the world. You are now safe in your quiet space with nothing but the abundance of positive energy.

Now, feel as your body accepts an abundance of energy from above, Feel it enter through the crown of your head, reaching down through your spine, being delivered to each fingertip. Feel it rush through you, as if you could not bear to handle another molecule of positivity.

Take another deep breath in and out. Focus your mind back on your energy capsule. Watch it glow and emanate with energy. Imagine now that it simply becomes invisible, unable to be seen by the naked eye, but there just the same.

Take this capsule with you for the rest of your day. It is your barrier to negativity, it will let nothing engulf your clear headspace. Imagine that the negative thoughts and *actions of others cannot penetrate this orb, it is your ultimate protection.*

Go about your day with infinite energy from the universe and an innate feeling of safety, as you are untouchable in your field of energy.

Use this guided meditation at any time to alleviate stress and re-center your focus on your inner self. Remember that the stress and negativity that you encounter on a daily basis can only affect you if you let themt in. Instead, make the conscious effort to create an aura of positive, protective energy all around you. With it, you are unstoppable.

Chapter 14: 30-Minute Complete Meditation

This complete meditation session is a great way to get started with your daily practice routine. While you may not have thirty minutes every day, spending a little more time in the early days of your practice may have more of a benefit. It can be difficult to calm the mind and get it to a relaxed, meditative state in a short time frame, and if you don't give yourself enough time, you might not see a big difference in your energy levels or apparent stress.

Try this routine any time you have the time to focus on the energy. We will use a combination of guided imagery and breathing techniques to revitalize mind, body, and spirit.

To begin, take a comfortable, seated position. Sit cross-legged, or in a comfortable way. Straighten your back so you are not slumped over, but do not strain your abdominal muscles or back. Simply be in a neutral, upright stance. Place your hands facing down upon your knees, or let them fall gently in your lap.

Take a deep breath in, filling your lungs to capacity. As you reach your limit, allow your exhale to take over, feel the air rushing out of your lungs. Take another deep breath, this time lingering in the fullness, before breathing back out. With every inhale, imagine that the breath is gathering your tension, and feel it leaving your body with each exhale.

Let us begin our breathing exercises. For this set, we will breathe in for a count of four, hold the breath for a count of six, then release for a count of eight. And begin.

In, two, three, four. Hold, two, three, four, five, six, out, two three, four, five, six, seven, eight.

On the last two beats of your exhale, feel the pressure as you push your abdominals to release every last bit of air. Imagine that this final push is releasing any stagnant air sitting idle at the bottom of your lungs. At this moment, it is making room for new, fresh air to be acquired, filling the body with new energy.

Complete this set of breathing another five to six times. Feel the energy coming in and out with each breath. Imagine it bringing in the fresh energy from around you, soaking every tissue and cell. Feel it seep on each finger and toe, feel them tingle with energy.

Now for a moment, just be with your breath. Do not count your breath, just let your chest rise and fall as it may. Just focus on the steady in and out of the breath. As you breathe in, don't force it, just let it reach its natural peak, then release.

Slowly move your right hand and place it over your heart. After a moment, place your left hand over your right, cupping over your heart area. Slow the breath, bow the head and simply sit with the beating of your heart. Feel it slow as you relax, bumping against your hand, happy and *healthy. Get the rhythm synced in your head, bump, bump, bump. Without much restriction, begin breathing in tune with this beat. Bump, bump, inhale, bump, bump exhale, along with the pattern of your breath.*

Now imagine that your heart sound fades quietly into the distance. It is not gone, just in the background, much like it always is. Now, feel the warmth of your skin on your palms as you gently return them carefully to your knees. Feel your bottom on the ground you sit on and imagine it transforming beneath you.

Feel the soft, warm sand as it cups your body, giving to every curve of your body. Wiggle your toes just slightly, feeling the grains of sand gather between your toes. Feel how warm the sun-kissed sand feels, warming your feet.

Imagine that you see in front of you a long, desolate beach. You sit silently, watching the sandy beach lessen and disappear along the horizon. It curves and abuts a grassy landscape to your left. You hear the light breeze move the parched grass, rustling. Deep within the grass, you hear the subtle chirping of sparrows. You cannot see them, but you can imagine them flitting about, gathering straw for their nests.

As you move your gaze slightly right, you see the dark blue water, crystal-like and fresh outspread all the way to the horizon. The waves are few away from shore, yet each one crashes with a force as it reaches the beach. As they come in slowly, one by one, you feel the bass of each one hitting the sand in your very core.

Imagine with each wave a great force of energy that has traveled far and wide across the sea. As it crashes on the beach, it becomes disheveled, yet gathers quickly. The energy has nowhere else to go but to you, the living creature who so desperately needs it.

Feel each crash like a jolt of energy awakening your body and soul. Feel it course through you, washing away any negative thoughts and emotions, neutralizing your fears.

As you sit with your new sense of power and positivity, feel the sun wash warmly over your shoulders. There is a calming warmth, despite the warm breeze that shields and surrounds you.

Smell the salt air coursing through your nostrils, entering deep into your lungs. Breathe in a big breath through your mouth, and feel the salt hit your taste buds. As you close your mouth, feel the light salt gather on your lips.

At this moment, all of your senses are engaged and an overwhelming sense of calm washes over you. There is nothing here in this moment to dwell on or get done, you are simply here on the beach, soaking in all of its ethereal energy.

Before leaving this place, make yourself a promise. From

this moment forward, carry this feeling in your heart. Remember the warmth of the sun on your shoulders, the soft sand beneath you. Feel the overwhelming coursing positivity flowing with each crash of the waves. Take this feeling with you as you depart back to the tasks of the day, and go forth with a renewed sense of purpose and wonder.

Take a deep breath, in all the way until your lungs are full, and breathe out slowly. As you breathe out, countdown slowly, three, two, one.

Open your eyes, harnessing the sense of powerful calm that has enveloped your mind and spirit. Take this feeling with you and depart in peace and happiness. This day shows great promise for you.

Conclusion

Thank you for making it through to the end of *Meditation for Beginners: Easy Guide to Begin Meditation*. Let's hope it was informative and able to provide you with all of the tools you need to achieve your goals of creating a daily meditative practice.

The next step is to identify a good time and place to include your practice. Be sure to give enough time to focus your mind and be optimistic about the outcomes of your practice. If one method does not speak to you, try something else.

In time, you will begin to reap the benefits of a daily meditative practice. Go forth with peace.

Finally, if you found this book useful in any way, a review on Amazon is always appreciated!

ALEX CHAND LEE

After a decade of stressful and hectic activity as professional stock trader, Alex overturned his lifestyle, returning to his ancient true passions: meditation, physical exercise and a simple and healthy lifestyle.
Hence the need to write, to direct those who have become overwhelmed by his same routine towards the rediscovery of a more "Humane" world, a world in which contact with nature and meditation become vital elements that draw the path to self-awareness and peace of mind.

www.ingramcontent.com/pod-product-compliance
Lightning Source LLC
Chambersburg PA
CBHW051917250726

48659CB00002B/693